Prader-Willi Syndrome

D0886180

The publication of this booklet was made possible through generous financial support by:

Swiss PWS Association

Foundation Growth Puberty Adolescence

and an unrestricted educational grant from Pfizer Endocrine Care.

Urs Eiholzer

Prader-Willi Syndrome

Coping with the Disease –
Living with Those Involved

68 figures, 57 in color, 2005

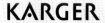

Basel • Freiburg • Paris • London • New York • Bangalore •
Bangkok • Singapore • Tokyo • Sydney

PD Dr. med. Urs Eiholzer
Institute Growth Puberty Adolescence
Möhrlistrasse 69
CH–8006 Zürich
Switzerland
www.childgrowth.org

Editing: Dr. Eberhard Zangger

All pictures are published with permission from the patients and their families, particularly with regard to printing them in their original form without masking the face. Copyright by Swiss PWS Association, c/o Dr. Andreas Bächli, President, Bugg 3, CH–9478 Azmoos (Switzerland).

Library of Congress Cataloging-in-Publication Data
A catalog record for this title is available from the Library of Congress.

Drug Dosage
The authors and the publisher have exerted every effort to ensure that drug selection and dosage set forth in this text are in accord with current recommendations and practice at the time of publication. However, in view of ongoing research, changes in government regulations, and the constant flow of information relating to drug therapy and drug reactions, the reader is urged to check the package insert for each drug for any change in indications and dosage and for added warnings and precautions. This is particularly important when the recommended agent is a new and/or infrequently employed drug.

© Copyright 2005 by S. Karger AG, P.O. Box, CH–4009 Basel (Switzerland)
www.karger.com
Printed in Switzerland on acid-free paper by Reinhardt Druck, Basel
ISBN 978–3–8055–7846–2 (English)
ISBN 978–3–8055–7845–5 (Deutsch)
ISBN 978–3–8055–8158–5 (Italiano)
ISBN 978–3–8055–8159–2 (Español)

Contents

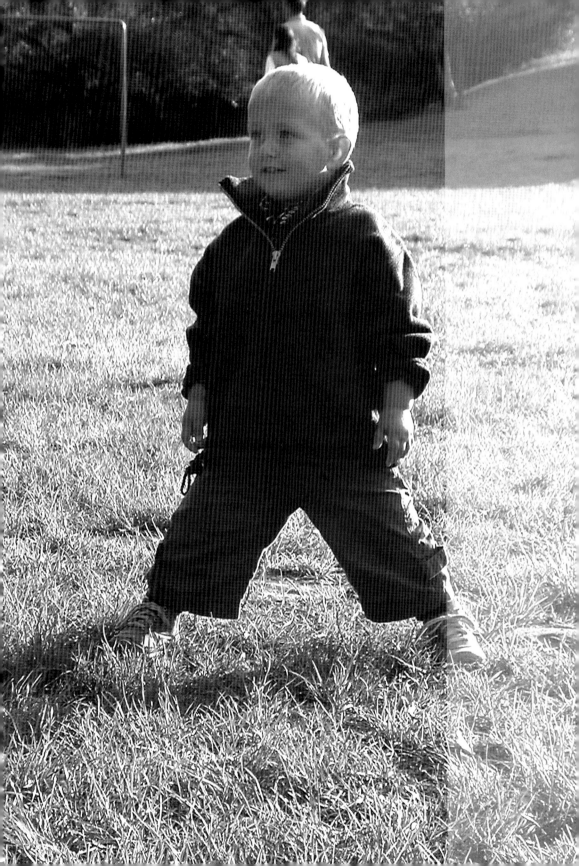

Everything's Different!

Our Child Is Born … Disabled

Joy and sorrow sometimes go hand in hand. Nobody knows that better than the parents of a disabled child. At first, when it becomes apparent that there might be something wrong with a newborn baby, they experience a growing sense of fear. Then comes the feeling of despair when it emerges that there really is something wrong. A clear diagnosis can bring enormous relief because the problem is given a name and an identity. However, when the parents begin to understand the diagnosis, fear takes over again. They start to imagine what it might mean for their future lives, their marriage and the development of the whole family. Finally comes the inevitable question 'Why us?'. Only then does the family begin to look forward and tackle the future.

With Prader-Willi syndrome (PWS), joy and sorrow continue to live side by side because the development of children with PWS is affected at all three levels: biological, psychological and social. Good times are frequently followed by difficult ones, with all the family's resources often stretched to the limit.

The aim of this booklet is to make life a little easier for parents, relatives, doctors and therapists of children with PWS by giving them a brief, comprehensible overview of what is currently known about this condition. The Swiss PWS Association first asked me to put something like this together a few years

'Of course it is important to know what PWS is and what the related problems are. But reports often forget to mention the "positive" side. Who of our friends, for example, could so easily take their baby to a restaurant without it constantly crying, as we can with our quiet Pierre? Most importantly, it is vital always to remember the joys you can experience with your child!'

ago. An initial edition was produced in 1998, based mainly on the experiences of parents from the Swiss PWS Association. In the last 5 years, however, research into appetite regulation in general as well as therapy for children with PWS have developed so much that it became necessary to revise the booklet completely and to make it internationally accessible by having it translated. I should point out that the latest scientific findings are also described in two comprehensive books which are currently available. Interested readers will find that they contain detailed information about topics which are only covered in general terms here. Despite – or perhaps because of – the tremendous progress in research on PWS, this booklet should be treated as a project which is permanently under construction rather than a finished product.

This publication is divided into six sections. After the introduction, the second chapter provides an overview of the history of research into the syndrome, its main characteristics and the most important methods of treatment. The third part describes the genetic causes, explains how the genetic defect is translated into the symptoms, and discusses the diagnostic process. The fourth and fifth sections contain detailed descriptions of the symptoms and methods of treatment, which are followed by a brief conclusion. In order to illustrate the everyday life of parents of children with PWS, we have added some excerpts from conversations with the parents of some of my patients.

I am grateful to Pfizer Endocrine Care and the Swiss PWS Association for its valuable suggestions and financial support for the publication of this booklet. I would also like to thank the Swiss National Foundation and the Swiss Academy for Medical Sciences, as well as the Pfizer, NovoNordisk and Serono companies for their long-standing support of our institute's research activities. I am particularly grateful to the Foundation Growth Puberty Adolescence and its board for its help and to my staff members – especially Dr. Dagmar l'Allemand, Michael Schlumpf and Claudia Weinmann – for their selfless contribution.

The most important share of my thankfulness goes to the children, adolescents and adults with PWS and their families, whose medical care I am in charge of. They enrich my daily life and I am thankful for being able to learn so much from them.

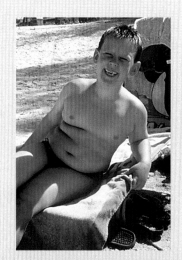
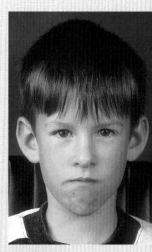
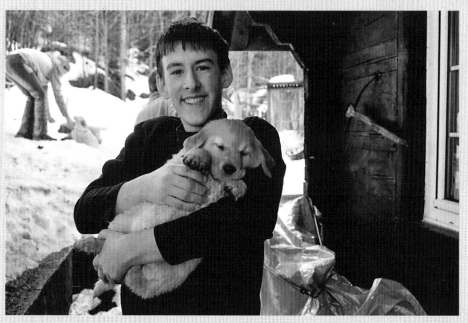

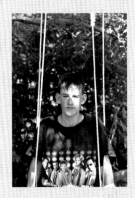

Marco

At nearly seven years, Marco started his weight reduction by intensive management, consistent control of food intake and growth hormone treatment. This turned the PWS child into a mostly normal boy. Marco practices as much sports as possible, in every possible way. As an adolescent, he lives through puberty as all the others of his age group and experiences its moments of happiness and thoughtfulness.

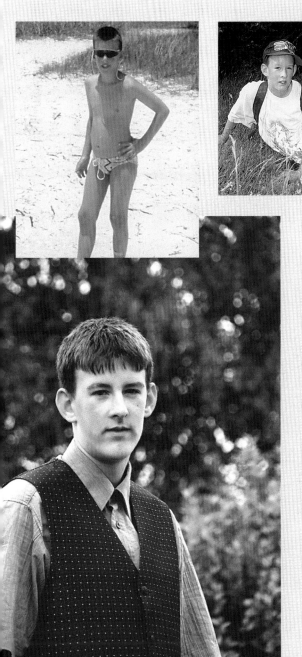

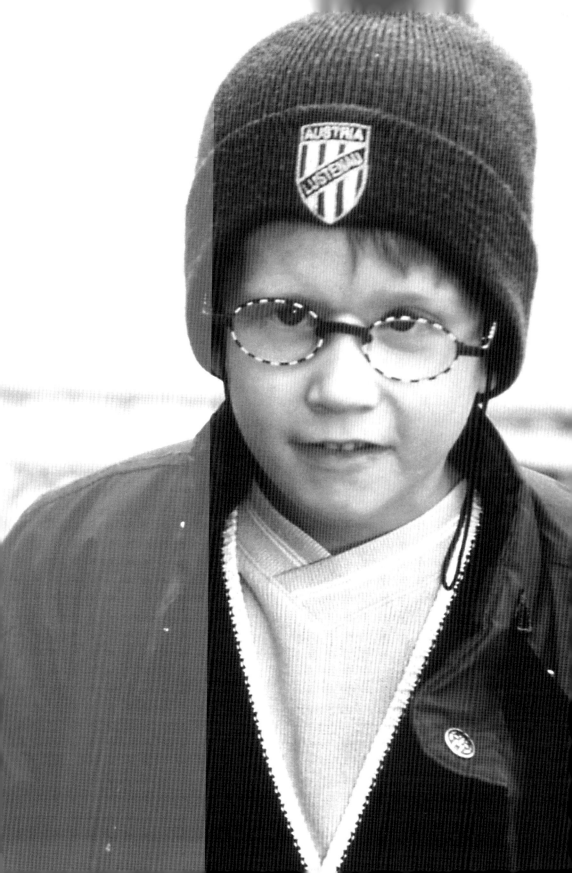

PWS –
An Overview

Research History

In the 1950s, Professor Andrea Prader, then head doctor at the Zurich Children's Hospital, noticed that he was repeatedly seeing children with similar symptoms: they were overweight, small in stature and often had small hands and feet and a low level of intelligence. In addition, these children's genitals were unusually small. Together with Professors Heinrich Willi and Alexis Labhart, Prader investigated these symptoms. In 1956, the three doctors were the first to describe Prader-Labhart-Willi syndrome, which nowadays is usually known as Prader-Willi syndrome, in a scientific publication.

What does the word 'syndrome' mean? How is it different from a disease? Whereas a disease has a clear, medically discernible cause, which leads to various symptoms, the symptoms of a syndrome, which often affect several organ systems, cannot be clearly traced back to a single cause.

Until 1981, the causes of PWS were unknown. The syndrome was only diagnosed on the basis of outward signs, such as short stature and obesity. [fig. 1] However, even back then doctors noticed that some cases exactly matched the description of Prader, Willi and Labhart, while in others the diagnosis was not quite so obvious.

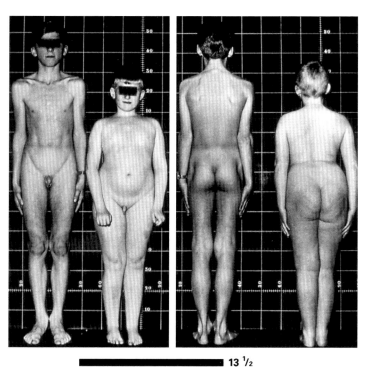

13 ¹/₂

[Fig. 1] Professor Prader had these 13-year-old twins photographed. The boy on the right clearly shows the classic symptoms of PWS: small stature, overweight with fat accumulation on the trunk (i.e. between shoulders and thighs), poorly developed genitals and scoliosis.

No explanation has yet been discovered as to why the severity of symptoms found in children with PWS varies so greatly. In terms of everyday life with a PWS child, this means one thing in particular: every child is different – every child needs different forms of help and individual support. This is why the assistance and advice of experts – specialists in different fields, speech therapists, nutritionalists, physiotherapists, orthopedagogues – are very important. The advice and experience of other parents of PWS children, which are equally helpful, can be exchanged through parents' support groups, for example.

Main Characteristics

Below is a summary of the most important characteristics of the syndrome. Many of them can nowadays be improved through special types of therapy.

Hypotonia

One of the earliest signs of PWS is hypotonia. Even in the womb, fetuses with PWS move less than healthy babies and, after birth, they lie virtually motionless. [fig. 2] As babies, their arms and legs appear weak and they move very little. They are very quiet, barely react to their environment and sleep a lot. Since hypotonia influences the ability to suck and swallow, PWS infants often do not get enough nourishment and become underweight. With time, the children get stronger and more alert, but a greater or lesser degree of muscle weakness still remains.

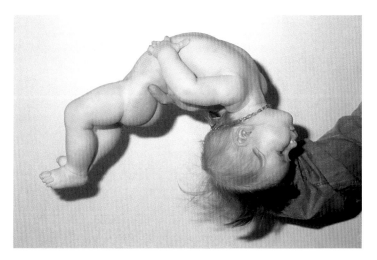

 [Fig. 2] 6-month old infant with PWS. Distinct hypotonia is typical for this age group. Healthy children in this position would normally keep their spine straight, head and legs pointing upwards.

Insatiable Appetite

Following these early problems of feeding and weight gain, the eating behavior of PWS children changes dramatically between the ages of 2 and 3. Eating becomes more and more impor- tant. [fig. 3] Later on, they virtually become addicted to food, a problem which remains with them more or less for the rest of their lives. Permanently monitoring and restricting food intake is the hardest yet most important task for parents and carers of children and adults with PWS. Unless clear boundaries are set

19

'Pierre's progress was slow. When he was about 6 weeks old, we could feed him with a bottle. However, we had to keep waking him up to feed because he never seemed to ask for it himself. Feeding sometimes took an hour – it was a real tightrope walk! At 6 months he started on solids and he could feed himself with a spoon after a year. He learned to sit and walk a good 6 months later than other children.'

from the beginning, the compulsion to eat leads to excessive weight gain and sometimes to severe obesity. Since PWS children are less active and mobile than other children, they also burn off fewer calories.

Short Stature

Another important feature of PWS is short stature. The stunted growth which can already be seen in infancy has its impact on adulthood: PWS patients remain small. Before the era of growth hormone therapy, the average height was 150 cm in women and 162 cm in men.

Hypogonadism

In children with PWS, underdeveloped genitalia can often already be seen at birth. In puberty, physical development is usually late in onset and incomplete. The voices of most young men with PWS do not break and most female PWS patients do not get their periods. They often have little interest in sex and a low sex drive. Because of their condition, people with PWS are usually infertile.

Mental Disability

The psychomotor and intellectual development of children with PWS is usually retarded from infancy. Speech and gross motor

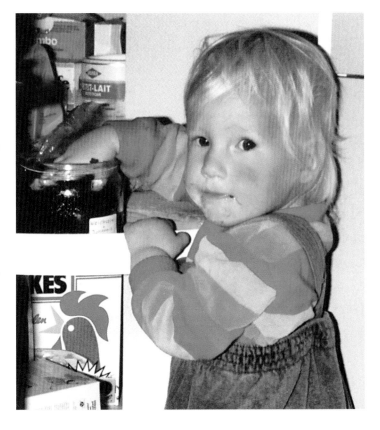

[Fig. 3] The change in eating behavior normally occurs between the age of two and four years – never overnight, but always gradually. If the children were given a choice of foods, they would prefer sweets and other food rich in calories.

skills (sitting, walking) are particularly affected. Although some children are able to attend normal schools, others clearly lag a long way behind children of the same age. Most feel more comfortable in smaller classes especially designed for children with educational needs.

Behavioral Problems

As babies, PWS children are usually good-natured and obedient. However, by school age they can sometimes become very difficult and throw uncontrollable temper tantrums. They are particularly upset by unexpected changes in their daily routine, as they like to know precisely and in advance what lies ahead. The tantrums, which many PWS children exhibit before puberty, become less common later on. However, some teenagers with PWS go through phases of depression, partly due to the fact that they gradually become more aware of being different.

It is difficult but very important for parents of PWS children to realise that, even with the best will in the world, they are not going to be able to 'cure' their child. The aptitudes of a child with PWS are established from birth. It is crucial that parents understand this, firstly so that they do not make excessive demands on their child and secondly so that they do not feel guilty. Even with constant therapy and excellent care, the limitations imposed by PWS cannot be overcome. At the same time, howev-

'At the age when children start to be awkward, Melanie had her first tantrums. These "attacks" are often triggered by unexpected changes to the daily routine, such as if Melanie has to come with me to visit someone at the last minute. There is often no clear reason for Melanie's screaming, door-slamming, etc. She will not be placated, even with patient explanations. Shouting back doesn't help either, so I usually send her to her room, where she quickly calms down.'

er, their awareness of these boundaries should not dishearten the parents and carers of PWS patients. Their input, combined with the support of a range of specialists, is vitally important for the patient's physical and mental well-being and is always worthwhile, even when the syndrome is not diagnosed immediately.

Main Forms of Treatment

The main difficulty with PWS is the sheer variety of the symptoms. Firstly, someone, such as the doctors in the maternity ward or, later on, the relevant pediatrician, needs to consider this diagnosis and have it confirmed. Usually, the case is automatically referred to a geneticist, who often explains the consequences of the diagnosis in detail to the parents. The parents then need a doctor who is familiar with the syndrome and who can explain the diversity of symptoms and create a relationship of trust. The doctor concerned should also be able to anticipate the specific problems caused by PWS and call in the various specialists at the right time in order to enlist their help. It is irrelevant which of the various specialists takes on this coordinating role. However, it is vital for the quality of life of the child concerned and his/her parents that this key function is fulfilled by a competent individual.

Restricting Calorie Intake

Controlling and restricting calorie intake was the first form of therapy that was used and remains the most effective means of weight management in PWS patients. The key to this treatment is to make sure that the patient receives the correct amount of food. Parents and teachers have to keep a close eye on all food, which is only possible if foods are strictly monitored and rigorously locked away. However, even such strict supervision can only limit and not prevent obesity.

Growth Hormone Treatment

Ever since the syndrome was discovered, short stature has been a known symptom of PWS. In the late 1980s, it was also discovered that PWS children have low muscle mass – in contrast to the muscle mass of most overweight children. Since small stature, increased fat mass and low muscle mass are all typical symptoms of growth hormone deficiency, children with PWS were first given growth hormone treatment in 1990. Several studies have shown that growth, body composition and physical performance can be significantly improved by growth hormone therapy. [fig. 4 a/b]

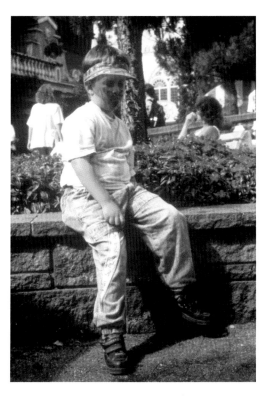

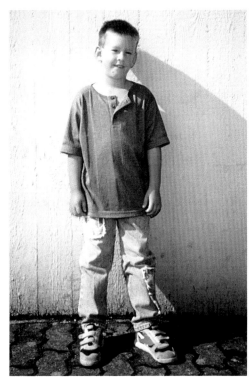

[Fig. 4 a/b] One of the first boys with PWS who was treated with growth hormone. Before treatment and after one year of therapy.

Daily Exercise

Inactivity and a lack of enthusiasm for physical exercise are also typical symptoms of PWS. Although growth hormone treatment can bring growth rates back to normal and improve body composition, the patient's muscle mass remains low and fat mass stays high, even if GH treatment is given over a long period and the patient's weight is normal. In order to improve muscle mass and increase energy consumption, it is sensible for the children and adults concerned to follow a structured daily exercise programme adapted to their own personal abilities and preferences. Parents, carers and PWS patients themselves need to be made very aware of the importance of physical activity. [fig. 5]

Sex Hormone Treatment

Incomplete pubertal development – for example, the fact that teenage boys' voices do not break – is very hard for PWS patients to cope with. The cause of this – hypogonadism (hypofunction of the testicles or ovaries) – is a central characteristic of PWS and affects not only pubertal development and psychological maturity, but also growth and body composition. Although hypogonadism is a well-documented symptom of PWS, sex hormone substitution is, to some extent, still a controversial therapy. This is related to the long-held belief that replacement with the male hormone testosterone can cause aggressive behavior in

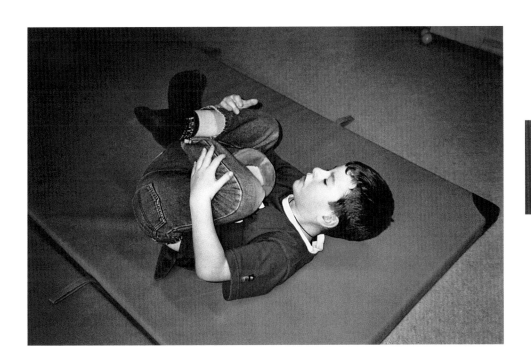

[Fig. 5] A 6-year-old during his daily physical exercise, which helps to improve muscle mass and increase energy consumption.

young men. The effects of puberty and sex hormone substitution on the behavior of PWS patients have never been scientifically investigated. We have always achieved good results through sex hormone substitution when such therapy has been started at the right time from a physiological point of view.

Early Support, Physiotherapy, Speech Therapy

Depending on the specific needs of the child and the types of therapy available locally, the necessary support is warranted from infancy. For the reason of the permanent hypotonia and low muscle mass, physiotherapy should primarily be aimed at strengthening the muscular system. Early support is designed to encourage the child to develop. If the child's speech development is delayed or impaired, it is important to seek the advice of a speech therapist at around the time of the child's third birthday.

Psychological Consultation

Families with PWS children are usually more prone to psychosocial problems than other families. It has also been shown that the style of upbringing can have a significant impact on the weight of children with PWS. Psychological counselling for parents or families is therefore designed firstly to support the people concerned and help them use their resources wisely and, secondly,

to help them bring up the child with greater clarity and consis-
tency. However, experience shows that families often find it hard
to admit that their own resources are no longer sufficient and
that they need outside help and support.

Pascal

As most children with PWS, when he was an infant, he was fed through a gastric feeding tube for a while, because due to his hypotonia, he was not able to suck properly. After his second birthday, Pascal's weight increased, even though his parents tried to limit his food intake. At the age of three, growth hormone therapy was instituted. Pascal is a happy child, even though he has to eat lots of vegetables and salads instead of french fries. Frequent physical activity is essential for improving muscle mass.

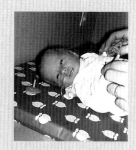

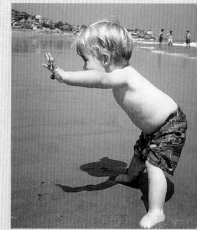

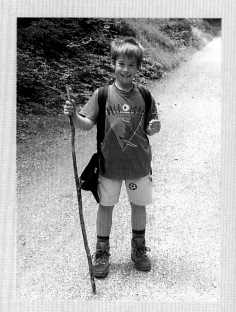

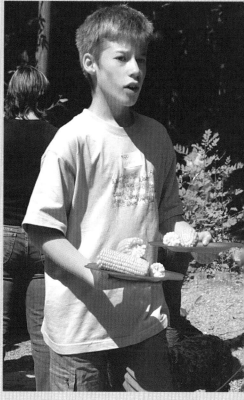

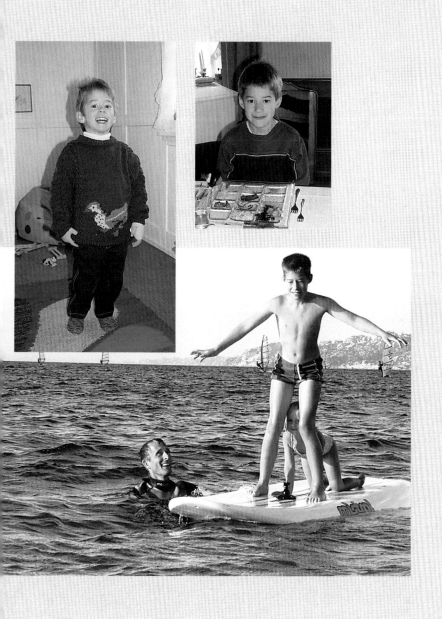

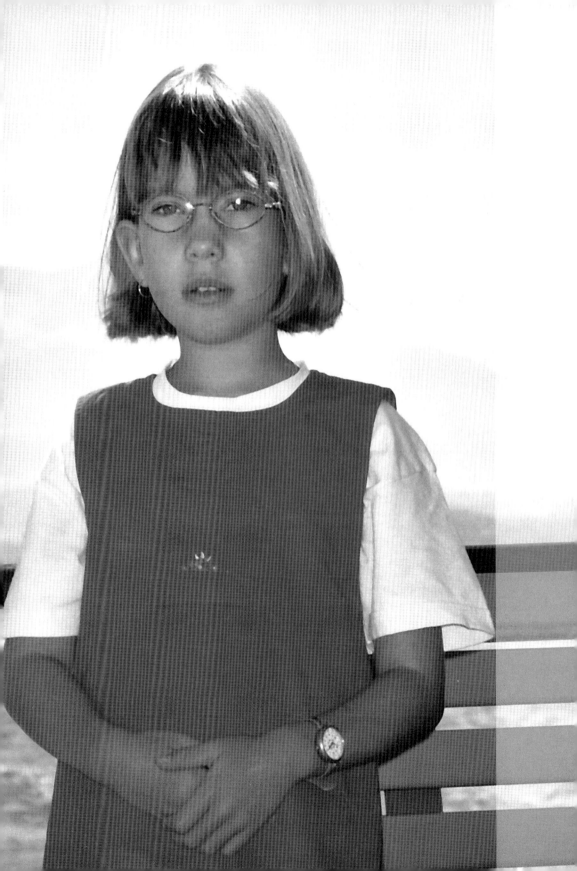

Genetic Causes and Diagnosis

PWS is caused by a chromosomal disorder. Chromosomes carry the genetic data we inherit from our parents. They store the information for all functions and predispositions of the human body. A chromosome is made up of two strands of protein (DNA strands), one short ('p') and one long ('q'). The two strands are joined together .

Every human cell contains a complete set of chromosomes, which is passed on every time a cell divides or multiplies. Each cell contains 46 chromosomes, two of which (the sex chromosomes) determine the person's gender. The other 44 chromosomes can be considered as 22 pairs, with both elements of each pair responsible for the same hereditary characteristic – one passed down from the mother and one from the father. In order to identify them, the 22 pairs of chromosomes are numbered 1 to 22 in order of size.

The actual genetic cause of PWS is now known. PWS always results when a piece of information on chromosome 15 inherited from the father is missing. This can occur in different ways:

1. In about 70% of people with PWS, there is a gap on the long strand of chromosome 15 inherited from the father (known as 'deletion' = loss of a small piece of the chromosome); in other words, the genetic information there is incomplete. If the deletion occurs on the maternal chromosome 15, the result is known as Angelman syndrome, a completely different condition which has nothing in common with PWS.

2. Most children with PWS who have no deletion on chromosome 15 have inherited both chromosomes 15 from their mother rather than one from each parent. This phenomenon – the transmission of two chromosomes from the same parent – is known as 'uniparental disomy'. It can occur either if, during the cell division that follows the fusion of the mother's egg cell and the father's sperm cell, both chromosomes from one parent fail to divide, or if an incorrect combination results from the re-joining process. In PWS cases, it is the two maternal chromosomes 15 that are passed on to the child; their structure is normal and the only 'mistake' is that they are wrongly distributed.

3. A small number of PWS children have neither a deletion nor uniparental disomy, but rather a so-called 'imprinting defect'. In these children, the 'imprinting center', in which the information is stored, is defective, irrespective of whether the chromosome concerned was inherited from the mother or the father.

All of these chromosomal abnormalities occur at the beginning of pregnancy. Such 'accidents' are normal in themselves, since even healthy human beings have many gaps in their chromosomes, but usually in places where the consequences are much less serious.

It can now be said that the genetic cause of the vast majority of PWS cases can be determined: the paternal information that should be carried in the long strand of chromosome 15 is faulty, either because the paternal chromosome 15 is incomplete (deletion), because it is missing altogether (uniparental disomy) or because the information that it was originally a paternal chromosome has been lost. Nevertheless, these discernible genetic defects do not quite account for all PWS cases – even today, a few cases have still not been explained.

Despite all these findings, it remains unclear how the genetic abnormality causes the symptoms of PWS. Research suggests that they are linked to a problem with the hypothalamus [see fig. 15], which controls such important functions as respiration, body temperature, sleep, appetite, activity, mood and even the endocrine system. The hypothalamus also plays an important role as the 'control center' for speech development and numerous other functions. The pituitary gland or hypophysis, which is also controlled by the hypothalamus, governs the body's other glands, which in turn regulate growth and pubertal development.

PWS is diagnosed using a DNA test on a blood sample, carried out in a genetic laboratory. Although this so-called 'methylation' test is not very expensive, it is extremely delicate and specific. If the test is positive, it is possible to identify the exact nature of the genetic abnormality through complex procedures.

If PWS is suspected, in other words if a baby has severe hypotonia or feeding problems, the methylation test should be carried out in the first few weeks if possible. Half of all infants with hypotonia actually have PWS. If the diagnosis is missed in infancy, it should be made at a later stage when the person concerned shows signs of obesity, delayed sexual development, insufficient growth, reduced intellect and other symptoms of PWS. Antenatal investigations are not generally carried out because virtually all patients are one-off cases with no family history of the syndrome. However, to be on the safe side, members of PWS families may be tested during pregnancy.

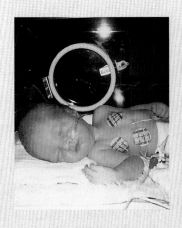

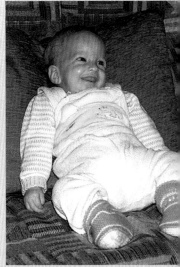

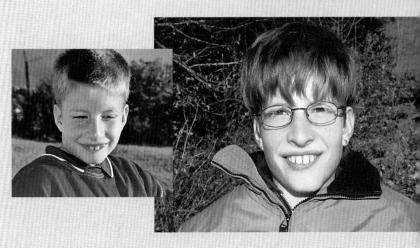

Manuel

Manuel too was fed through a gastric feeding tube during the first weeks.
Manuel was probably the first child ever that received growth hormone
treatment at the age of two years. Frequent sports activities and consistent
dietary control promote his excellent physical development. Manuel is very
concentrated when he does his homework with joy and dedication. He is
almost a child like any other.

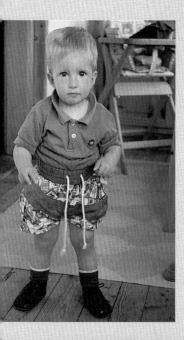
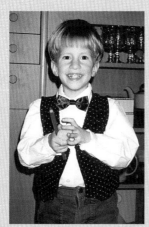
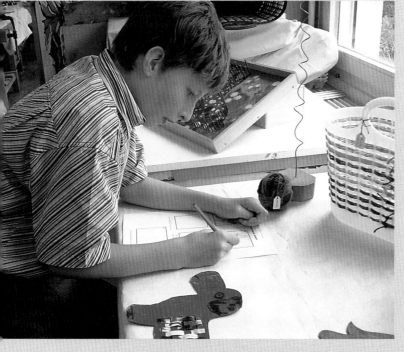

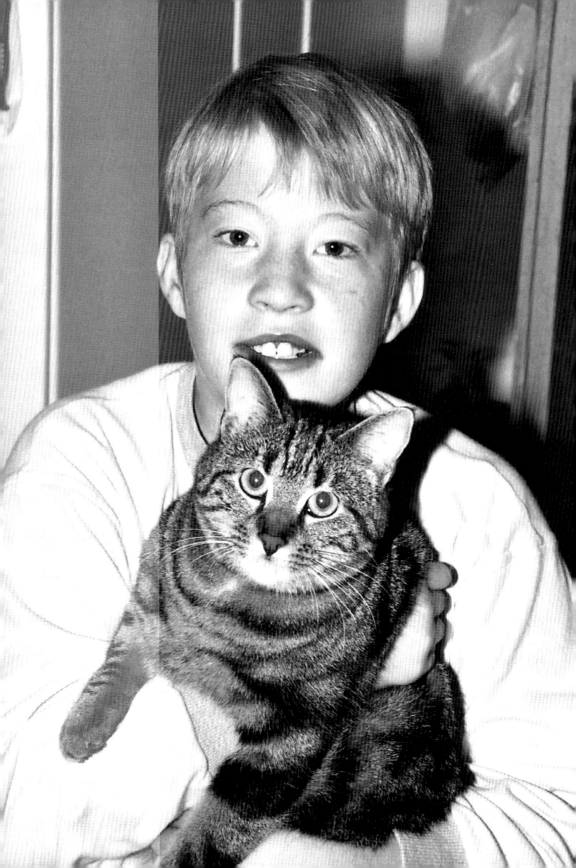

Symptoms

All the symptoms described below are typical of PWS. However, they affect each person with PWS to differing degrees. Some physical symptoms, such as hypotonia or reduced growth, can be recorded objectively. However, the emotional and intellectual development of children with PWS is more difficult to characterise; each child is different, learns differently and progresses differently.

Hypotonia

Severe hypotonia is one of the first signs of PWS. It is often evident before birth, since babies with PWS move less in the womb than other children. Therefore, they often do not turn into a suitable delivery position, but lie in the breech position, which can sometimes necessitate a Caesarean section.

Hypotonia usually becomes obvious immediately after birth. It is the main symptom of PWS in the first year of life. PWS children sleep a lot and barely move their weak arms and legs. They often have to be woken to feed and are quite likely to fall asleep again while feeding. Hypotonia also affects the ability to suck and swallow and infants cannot suck hard enough to take in sufficient nourishment. This makes breastfeeding difficult and leads to nutrient deficiencies. Even bottle-feeding takes a

'Stefan was very quiet. In contrast to my previous pregnancies, I could feel him moving much less. Just before he was born, he turned into the breech position. Since I was a few days past my due date, they put the tocograph on. Stefan kept going to sleep and had to be woken up through the abdominal wall. I was having contractions but there was no progress. In the end, they performed a Caesarean.'

'As soon as she was born, we realised that Melanie had severe hypotonia. Her arms and legs were all floppy, she was all limp as if she had no bones. She couldn't cry properly, it sounded more like a whimper or a quiet whistle. She had problems maintaining her body temperature and had to spend two days in an incubator. She also was not strong enough to drink and was therefore fed through a tube into her stomach for the first few days. I could not breastfeed her because she could not suck hard enough. However, a bottle with a large teat hole worked. We were allowed to take her home a week after she was born.'

long time. Sometimes a special teat with a larger opening can help, but because the baby's swallowing reflex is not adequately developed, there is a risk of choking. Many children with PWS therefore have to be fed through a tube for a while.

Since they are initially undernourished, infants with PWS are often underweight in their first few weeks of life and grow less quickly than healthy babies of the same age. Most remain motionless, sleep a lot and barely react to their environment. They rarely cry, but when they do, they do so very quietly. [fig. 6]

Muscle tone improves over time, so PWS children can then drink more and put on weight. They become stronger and take an interest in their surroundings: they laugh, enjoy attention and stimulation and, because they hardly cry, are lovable and easy to look after. [fig. 7] Even when they are ill they rarely cry, which can be because some children with PWS have a higher pain threshold and develop fevers less quickly than other children. Illnesses can therefore sometimes be hard to detect.

Although they become stronger and more attentive, PWS children's muscle tone remains weak and they show little desire to move at all, let alone romp around. Alongside hypotonia, this

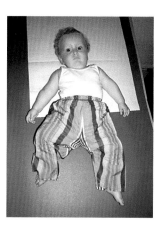

[Fig. 6] Infants with PWS move little, sleep a lot and participate only little in what is going on around them.

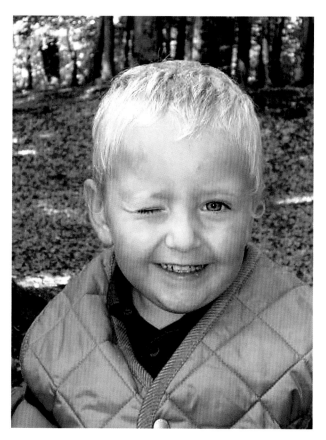

[Fig. 7] In children, muscle mass is improved, they laugh more often and enjoy the attention that they are given.

'Jeremy could walk at 16 months and ride a tricycle at 3 years of age. But he had to put an enormous effort into achieving these things. In the first 2 years, we went to the physiotherapist four times a week and practised a lot at home as well. Jeremy joined a play group when he was four and a half and that did him good. It was important for him to become more independent of his mother and to mix with other children. For he often had no desire to move around.'

is partly due to a poor sense of balance: climbing, riding a bicycle and sliding down banisters all require balance and strength. Sometimes, a PWS child might fall asleep while playing. On the other hand, many PWS children frequently wake up at night. Many play quite happily for a while before going back to sleep.

'The more mobile Melanie became, the more she would go hunting for food. I remember how she stood on tiptoe and pulled the bread off the stove and how she went for the jam in the fridge. At the beginning, she was still slim and we watched with some amusement. At nursery school, she started eating the bread other children had brought.'

Weight and Energy Balance

Parents of children with PWS have to deal with feeding problems shortly after the birth, although initially they are the opposite of later problems. As infants, PWS children are underweight. At this stage, the desire for them to put on weight is the main concern for their parents and the doctors looking after them. It is important to feed infants and babies well and to find the time to do this. When PWS is diagnosed early on, many parents are so worried about their child's anticipated obsession with food that they do not feed their child enough in the first few years and thereby aggravate their growth problems. The risk is heightened by the fact that PWS infants tend to remain quiet and do not scream when they are hungry. It is therefore helpful for parents to consult a nutritional adviser early on in order to find out how much their child should be eating and drinking each day if they are to achieve optimal nourishment.

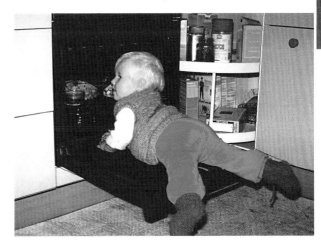

[Fig. 8] The change in eating behaviour usually sets in at an age between two and four years. It never occurs overnight, but always gradually. The girl is crawling into the oven to get to the fresh bread, since she is not yet able to walk properly.

All parents whose child has been diagnosed with PWS know that, at some point, their child is going to develop an enormous appetite. The change in eating behavior usually begins between the ages of two and four and does not occur overnight, but gradually. This transformation is extremely confusing for the parents, who are naturally concerned about their child's eating habits. Is the child really over-eating? Is his/her appetite under control? Consulting a nutritional expert can also be very helpful at this stage.

The constant urge to eat causes PWS children to become massively overweight if nothing is done to stop it. They particularly love to eat sweets and other high-calorie foods. They will try to get hold of them whenever possible, sometimes employing very cunning ways of doing so. [fig. 8] Since children with PWS are less active and enthusiastic about movement than other children, they also burn off fewer calories. The weight increase that results from the imbalance between excessive eating and reduced energy consumption serves only to dissuade them from exercising even further – a vicious circle. Body fat mainly tends to develop around the thighs, upper arms, abdomen and buttocks, while the lower arms and legs remain slim. Obesity is all the more obvious since children with PWS grow slowly and not very tall.

The reason for the constant need to eat is a disordered satiety function. This is probably the result of a hormone imbalance, although this has not yet been clearly identified. It is thought that one or more signals which indicate satiety do not reach the hypothalamus in people with PWS, so that they never feel full and must always be on the lookout for food. Despite their increased fat mass, their brain tells them that they are always hungry and need to eat constantly. The main energy control point in the hypothalamus does not detect the energy reserves available (the excess fatty tissue), but only sends out the message 'keep eating'. Healthy people find it hard to imagine such a feeling of hunger, but it should not be underestimated. It can totally govern the thoughts and actions of persons with PWS. [fig. 9]

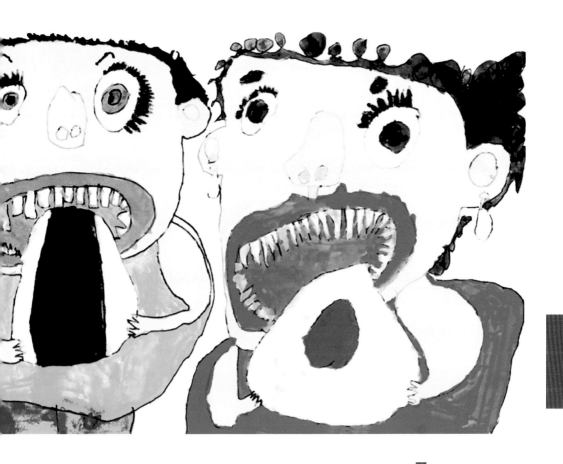

[Fig. 9] Drawing by the
7-year-old Hirotaka.
It shows his mother and
his insatiable appetite.

Outside help from doctors and nutritional advisers can take some of the burden off the parents where eating is concerned. Psychological counselling is also helpful in relation to the monitoring and limitation of the child's food intake. This adjustment of eating habits also has an impact within the family: everyone, including parents, brothers and sisters, must abide by certain agreed rules with regard to eating, such as fixed meal times and carefully measured portions. Siblings must not spoil their brother or sister by giving them extra portions or sweets. The whole family must adapt to the exceptional abilities of PWS children to obtain food. In most cases, even the fridge and kitchen cupboards have to be locked. Parents must also bring their child up without using food as a reward.

Since children with PWS enjoy eating and will put anything in their mouths, they are particularly at risk – as are all small children – from poisonous substances in the house and garden. Medicines, cleaning equipment, paint, etc. must be locked away and a close eye kept on poisonous plants in the garden.

As they grow older, new problems arise as the children come into contact with other people: neighbours, friends at nursery and school, teachers and relatives must be made aware that the parents are not stopping their child from eating through maliciousness, but out of necessity. Informing other people be-

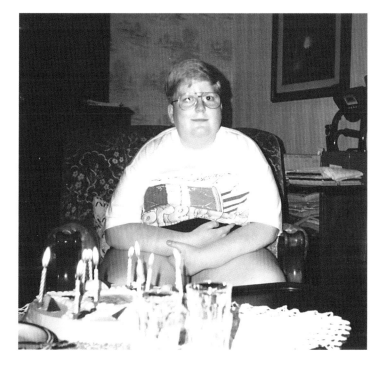

 [Fig. 10] An adolescent with PWS before the growth hormone era.

'Jeremy, even now at the age of 10, is really bone idle. He is happiest sitting down. He can spend hours doing puzzles, watching TV or just gawping at what's going on around him.'

comes very important. As they get older, the children themselves can also understand why they have to watch what they eat. However, the need to eat will triumph more and more often over the desire to please the parents (by not eating). People with PWS therefore need their food intake to be controlled throughout their lives by their carers in order to prevent obesity. [fig. 10]

Reduced Activity Levels

Researchers still do not know exactly why children with PWS are so prone to obesity. It is clear, however, that their sense of satiety is underdeveloped and that they could therefore eat endlessly unless someone stops them. It is nonetheless also evident that PWS children burn the same amount of calories as other chil-

'At first we couldn't understand why we had to be strict about Stefan's calorie intake because, when he was a baby, we rejoiced with every drop he drank. However, he put on weight very quickly between the ages of three and four and we realised we had to be careful. Since then, his eating has settled down really well. Stefan, like his brothers and sisters, has to ask when he wants something to eat. In order to be able to give him seconds if necessary, we give Stefan only half a portion on his plate and make sure he has plenty of vegetables or salad. Recently, he has secretly pinched some bread several times. But so far we have not had to lock the food cupboards and fridge. Adults cause the most problems: some friends and neighbors simply cannot understand why Stefan can't eat biscuits between meals, for example. We have tried to tell them why, but it makes no difference. We have sometimes therefore resorted to a white lie and told people he is diabetic – that has helped.'

dren when they exercise. However, they move around much less than healthy children, which is another cause of obesity. Their body composition is therefore different from that of other overweight children, who have above-average fat tissue, but also more muscles to transport their heavy bodies. Children with PWS, in contrast, have fewer muscles in spite of their high fatty tissue levels. It recently became clear that the main reason children with PWS have fewer muscles is because they move less. More movement means more muscles and more muscles burn off more fat. A special exercise programme lasting 10 min each day, for example, can therefore help keep their weight down. [fig. 11]

Short Stature

Delayed growth is noticeable from infancy. PWS children continue to grow slowly and, as adults, are much smaller than most people. On average, women reach a height of 150 cm and men 162 cm. Unlike other children, they do not experience a growth spurt during puberty. However, PWS children with tall parents grow taller than those from 'smaller' families.

It is now thought that the delayed growth of children with PWS is caused by a growth hormone deficiency. Growth hormone is formed in the pituitary gland and distributed through

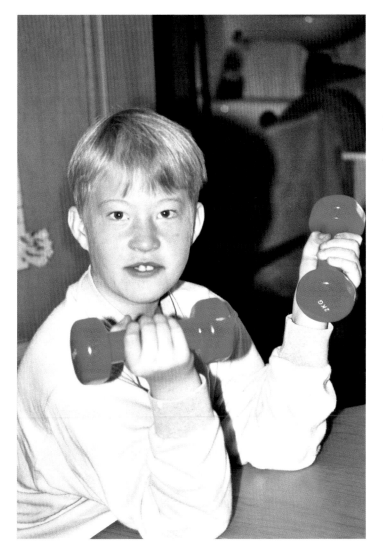

[Fig. 11] Daily physical exercise helps children with PWS to build more muscles and thus to burn more energy.

the body in the bloodstream. It is controlled by a region of the intermediate brain, the hypothalamus. Growth hormone not only provides the impulse for growth, but also promotes muscle formation and strength and reduces the production of fatty tissue.

Generally speaking, there may be many different reasons for a growth hormone deficiency. For example, the pituitary gland may fail to produce any or enough growth hormone from birth onwards. Alternatively, the pituitary gland may be damaged later on by an accident or tumor. In some cases, hormone production and transport are fine, but the body does not respond to the growth impulse. With PWS, the pituitary gland probably works perfectly well, but the way it is controlled by the hypothalamus is defective.

Sexual Development

At birth, many children with PWS have underdeveloped genitals. In males, the penis has a normal structure but is often very small. In females, the small lips of the vulva and clitoris are often underdeveloped. In boys, one or both testes may be undescended. Neither the testes nor the scrotum are fully developed. This is probably due on the one hand to the generally poor muscle tone of children with PWS and, on the other, to the low level of sex hormone production in the testes before birth, which is related to inadequate regulation by the pituitary gland and hypothalamus.

The question of undescended testes is clearly closely linked to subsequent fertility. It is assumed that boys with PWS are infertile because sperm cells can only be formed through precise regulation by the hormones released by the pituitary gland. This in turn must be accurately controlled by the hypothalamus. Since this control is defective in people with PWS, male patients appear highly unlikely to be fertile.

Also concerning puberty, children with PWS are different from other children. In most cases, the sex hormone deficiency means that puberty more or less does not happen, especially in boys, who often show only slight pubertal development. Their voices often do not break. Most girls develop further, but the majority never reach full sexual maturity. Some do not experience menstruation at all, while at the other end of the spectrum, a very small number do have regular periods. In such cases, fertility and the possibility of pregnancy cannot be ruled out. Across the world, only two women with PWS have been known to fall pregnant and give birth to healthy children.

Psychomotor Development and Intelligence

Children with PWS suffer from reduced psychomotor and intellectual development, which is evident from infancy. Often, the development of speech and gross motor skills is particularly slow. Many children have difficulty learning to talk, although their understanding of language is often better. Most PWS patients have severe learning difficulties, with an average IQ of 70. However, intelligence levels cover the whole IQ spectrum, so some people with PWS have a normal level of intelligence. The diversity is as broad as with healthy children. However, because of behavioral problems and difficulties with specific tasks, even those with normal intelligence are likely to experience problems at school. Some children with PWS are capable of attending a normal school, although most feel more at home in small classes, where they can learn at their own pace and their own personal strengths can be developed.

'Anja has now caught up to some extent, but she is still a disabled child. This is obvious because we can compare her every day with her twin brother: he can now walk, whereas Anja has only just started crawling. Our son can string together a four-word sentence while Anja can only say individual words in a squeaky, nasal voice.'

Social Development and Behavior

People with PWS also experience problems with their social development. They have difficulty evaluating social situations correctly. In some circumstances, speech and language problems can make matters even worse.

As babies and toddlers, children with PWS are sweet and loving. However, as they get older and start testing their boundaries, they can react very violently and defiantly, often with fits of rage. The cute, obedient toddler can turn into an extremely stubborn child who slams doors and is virtually impossible to calm down.

The mood of a PWS child can change very quickly. Many are particularly upset by unexpected changes to their daily routine, since they like to know precisely and in advance what lies ahead. An imminent event has to be talked through again and again and the child can ask the same question a thousand times. If this strategy fails, tantrums may result. Many children dig their heels in and carry on as normal. However, they are often very trusting and express their feelings – both positive and negative – quite openly.

'If we ever said no to Monika, she reacted by screaming loudly, throwing things around, flinging herself to the floor and generally going crazy. These outbursts happened until she was around nursery school age. In the last few years she has become more able to deal with frustration and can cope fairly well with sudden changes of plan. Of course we try to change our plans as little as possible at the last minute. However, when we have done so, we have tried to get her used to the new situation and explain the positive sides as much as possible. In the meantime, she has developed her own strategies for coping with such changes.'

It is a mystery why this phase of defiance is often more pronounced among PWS children than with others. However, parents' experience suggests that, as well as being an age-related phenomenon, the anger and despair are often related to the need for everything to be planned in advance. Anything which upsets the prescribed order of events confuses the child, who reacts with anger and defiance.

It can therefore be helpful if parents prepare their children in advance for changes to their schedule, emphasise the positive aspects of the new plan, talk about difficult situations before they arise and maybe even act them out as role-plays. However, it is also important that children with PWS are taught at an early age to be flexible, as this will make change easier to cope with. Flexibility can be taught in small, everyday situations. For example, a child can learn to choose between two possibilities, such as which clothes to wear.

If the child still has a tantrum, attempts to talk or argue with them rarely improves the situation and sometimes even aggravates it. It is often wiser to leave the room or to send the child to their bedroom until they have calmed down.

When they first go to nursery or school, their sphere of activity grows and they become more independent. This makes them proud, but also creates new problems. On the one hand, the compulsive obsession with finding food away from the home can lead to weight gain. Generally speaking, as the child becomes more independent, it becomes harder to keep their weight at a reasonable level. On the other hand, PWS children become more aware of their disability when they spend time with children of the same age. Nursery and school-age children with PWS sometimes suffer just because they are different, which can also lead to uncontrollable outbursts of rage. Parents can do nothing to stop their children feeling excluded. However, together with nursery-school and school teachers, they can help to build up the child's self-esteem. Praise is just as useful as working together to develop strategies on how to deal with frustration.

After puberty, reactions of defiance and tantrums become less common, although bouts of depression are more likely and are sometimes accompanied by psychotic symptoms. Here also it is important that the people concerned are taken seriously and that their self-esteem is boosted. A structured environment is very helpful for all PWS patients. It can also be useful to learn behavioral techniques, to attend psychotherapy sessions (possibly in a group) and, in some cases, to take psychiatric drugs.

Many children with PWS have their own sleep patterns, dropping off now and again during the day and waking up at night. During the day, parents and teachers should wake the child if they fall asleep so that they develop a regular wake/sleep routine. As they grow older, waking up at night becomes less of a

'At first, Jeremy went to a normal nursery school with 28 children. He could also have gone to a normal primary school, but our experiences at nursery showed us that a smaller group was better for him. Because if he constantly has to measure himself against others and thinks he is not keeping up, he retreats into his shell or has tantrums. We therefore put Jeremy in a small class.'

problem. With a bit of explanation and a more established routine, older children who wake up at night can learn to play by themselves until they go back to sleep. However, some parents have discovered that their children go looking for food in the house when they wake up at night, which clearly goes against all dieting plans.

'Susanne is now 26. She has done a two-year housekeeping course and now she spends the week in a residential home, where she works in the kitchen. In her spare time, she loves writing letters, playing the flute and listening to music. She spends weekends either with her family or with the parents of her two friends. She is very strict with herself about her weight: she weighs herself every day and, if she has put on weight, she cuts back on what she eats and skips her afternoon snack, for example. She enjoys spending the holidays outdoors, camping.'

Respiratory Problems

It has been known for a long time that some children with PWS have respiratory problems. [fig. 12] This can be due to various causes: sometimes regulation by the hypothalamus is abnormal and not quite at the usual level; reduced muscle mass can lead to inadequate respiratory movements; and sometimes the anatomy of the throat is narrow in PWS children, resulting in restricted air flow. It is important that such situations are recognised early, particularly if the child snores at night or sometimes stops breathing. [fig. 13] A polygraph is usually obtained in such cases. This involves the child spending a night in hospital so that breathing, heart-rate and brain functions can be measured. They are also examined by an ear, nose and throat specialist who should check whether their tonsils are enlarged or not. Enlarged tonsils are very common in PWS and should be removed as quickly as possible.

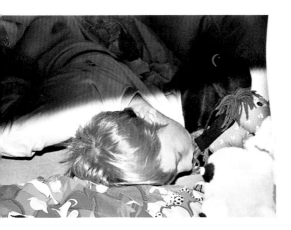

[Fig. 12] To illustrate the respiration problem: A sleeping girl who bends her neck backwards thus instinctively giving the airways a maximum of space.

Orthopedic Problems

Children with PWS are more likely than other children to suffer from curvature of the spine. Here again, the parents need to be vigilant, because they are likely to be the first to notice a change in their child's posture. Depending on the extent and seriousness of the case, physiotherapy or, in rare cases, treatment with a corset may be necessary. Since any curvature of the spine (forwards = kyphosis; lateral = scoliosis) increases as the child grows, it must be continuously monitored, particularly during periods of rapid growth (for example, in the early stages of growth hormone treatment). If in doubt, the doctor responsible will seek the advice of an orthopedic specialist.

Dental Problems

Good dental hygiene is important for all children. However, since the teeth of PWS children are often worn down more quickly because the enamel is less robust, they need to be cared for and monitored particularly closely. Furthermore, the saliva of children with PWS is thicker than that of other children, which means they often have dried saliva at the corners of their mouth. Thick saliva does not protect the teeth from decay as effectively

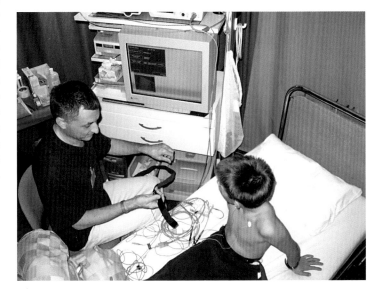

[Fig. 13] A doctor explains the sleep examination (polysomnography) to a child with PWS. For this examination, the children spend one night in the hospital, where respiration, heart rate and brain function are recorded.

as normal, thinner saliva. The eating habits of children with PWS, particularly their love of sweet foods, increase the risk of decay even further. Therefore, they should regularly see a dentist from around the age of three at the latest. It is worth finding a child-friendly dentist who is able to put the child at ease and therefore reduce the risk of tantrums.

Skin Problems

Children with PWS tend to scratch insect bites and lesions with particular vigour. Since this not only delays the healing process but also can lead to infection, it is sensible to take simple measures to counter the problem. These might include ointments and creams which reduce the itching; short fingernails can also limit scratching. Educating the child about the effects of scratching can also help give lesions and bites time to heal, as the child learns to scratch around the lesion or rub it with their hand rather than scratching it with their fingernails. Parents of children with PWS also report that regular stimulation with a massage brush reduces the urge to scratch. However, if a deep lesion has been caused by a lot of scratching, it will need to be treated carefully, often with local antibiotics and, most importantly, with a firm bandage to stop the child scratching it even more.

Matthias

Matthias was the first child ever that received consistent and comprehensive management and growth hormone therapy from the age of seven months on. He not only attends one hour per week of physiotherapy, but is consistently encouraged to physical exercise by his family. In combination with consistent food intake control this results in a favorable muscle-fat ratio. Matthias is happy. When he plays or at official events (first Communion), he can hardly be told apart from healthy children.

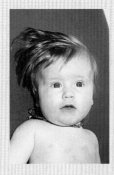

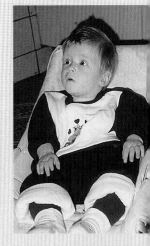

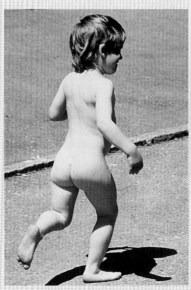

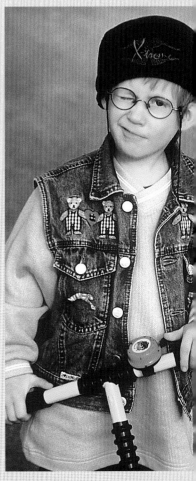

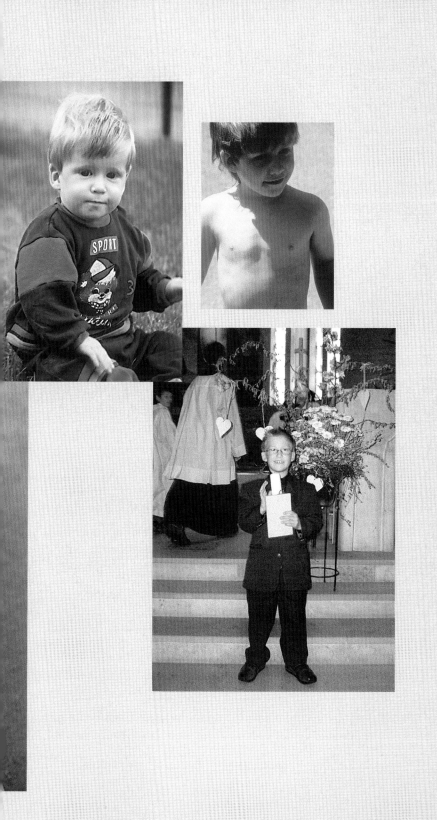

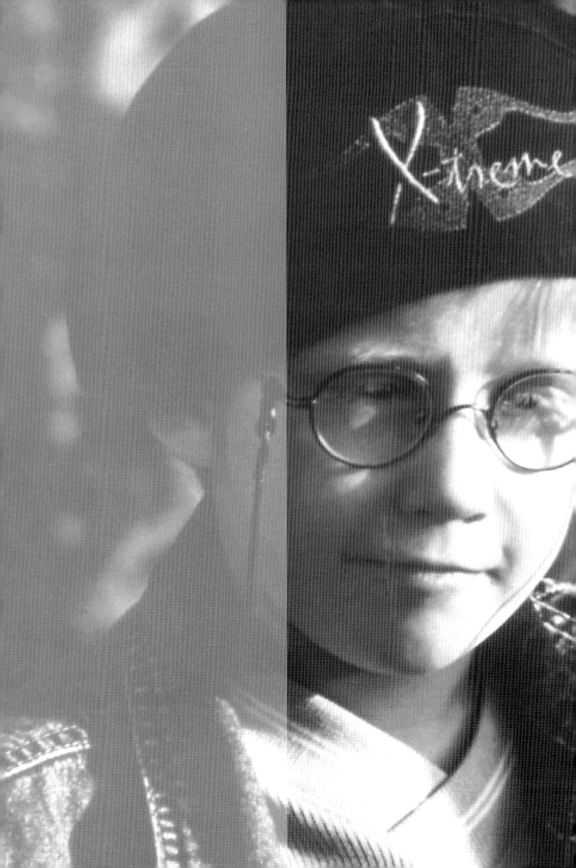

Treatment Strategies

Limiting Food Intake and Regulating Appetite

Limiting calorie intake is and remains the most important task for anyone looking after a child with PWS. Older children, adolescents and adults with PWS need to keep the kitchen and fridge locked. In order to prevent obesity, it is paramount to control the child's eating habits before they become overweight. Professional nutritional advice either from a doctor very experienced in PWS or a nutritional expert is usually essential. It is important to ensure that, although they do not need large amounts of food, children with PWS are given a balanced diet, including sufficient calcium, trace elements and vitamins. The support of a suitably experienced psychologist can also be useful, since parents often know all there is to know about nutritional matters but have trouble implementing it. It has also been proven in recent years that children with PWS need to not only restrict their energy intake (by controlling their eating) but also to use more energy (through movement and sport). For children with PWS not only eat too much, they also move around much less than healthy children.

If more energy is ingested in the form of food than is burnt off through movement, i.e. if input exceeds output, then fat

'The whole family's eating habits changed: we never eat between meals and if my eldest daughter wants some sweets she is not allowed to eat them in front of Anja. We make sure there is nothing edible within Anja's reach. Anja's grandmothers think we are too strict with her, but we are sure it is worthwhile being consistent. We have already had one success. At a birthday party, the table was full of cakes and sweets – but Anja helped herself to a tomato!'

reserves begin to build up. A perfectly functioning energy regulation system and sufficient energy storage are fundamentally important for all living things, since energy intake and consumption usually take place at different times: we rest and eat and only later do we start moving again. Many animals put on an extra layer of fat in the autumn to see them through the winter. Even human beings used to do something similar, putting on extra fat when times were good in order to survive the next famine. Energy consumption also varies tremendously. People use up very few calories at their desks, but a lot more if they run a marathon.

Unless their eating is controlled, PWS patients often weigh over 100 kg, or even up to 300 kg in extreme cases. Of course it would be wrong to want to make PWS children skinny. Our aim is to keep their weight at a reasonable level in relation to their height, i.e. between the 75th and 97th percentiles on the chart. [fig. 14] In our experience, people with PWS in this sector of the chart have the optimal muscle/fat ratio.

Medicines used by non-PWS overweight people to regulate their appetite appear to have no effect on the constant hunger and weight gain experienced by PWS patients. Psychiatric drugs that are used to treat depression or other problems appear to have no impact on eating behavior.

Growth Hormone Therapy

Towards the end of the 1980s, researchers realized that children with PWS might suffer from a growth hormone deficiency. Growth hormone is produced in the pituitary gland and controls growth as well as other biological processes such as muscle formation and the burning of fat. The pituitary gland hangs on a stalk underneath the brain and is controlled by hormones produced by the hypothalamus. [fig. 15] Children who – usually due to a congenital defect – are born without a pituitary gland cannot produce growth hormone and therefore do not grow properly. In addition, they develop fewer muscles and more fatty tissue than healthy children. They therefore display similar symptoms to children with PWS: insufficient growth, obesity, reduced muscle tissue. However, they tend to be less overweight than children with PWS.

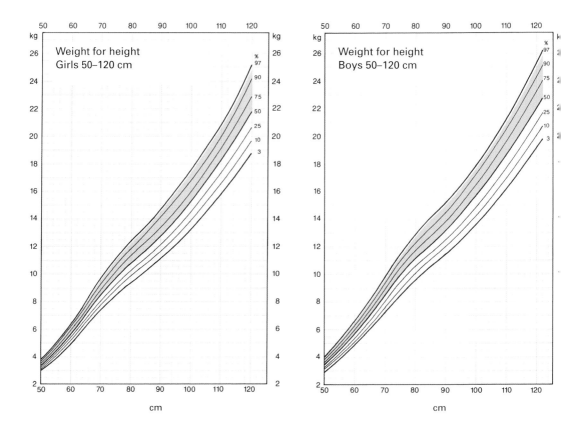

Since it is particularly hard to prove that an overweight child has a growth hormone deficiency, it took a long time for people to realise that most children with PWS actually do not produce sufficient growth hormone. Overweight people have a low growth hormone level compared to people with normal

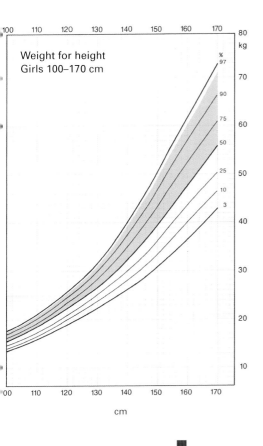

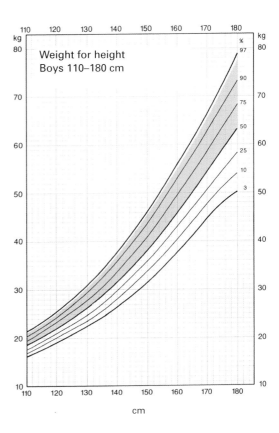

[Fig. 14] Centile graphs to depict weight in relation to height. The 50th centile corresponds to the average body weight of healthy children. The area between the 3rd and 97th centile is defined as normal range. Only 3% of all children have a weight below the 3rd centile, and only 3% above the 97th centile. For children with PWS, the optimum weight range lies between the 50th and 95th centile.

These centile graphs are available as PDF documents: www.childgrowth.org

Info box:

Leptin, Insulin and Other Tools of Hunger Regulation

Many biological systems are safeguarded in several different ways. This also applies to energy regulation. We currently know a little about this system. It has been discovered that energy is regulated via two independent mechanisms – one which actively produces hunger and one which stops hunger.

In 1995, leptin, a hormone produced by fat cells, was discovered. The more fatty tissue a person has, the more leptin they have in their blood. The same applies to insulin, which is produced by the pancreas. The more fatty tissue a person has, the higher their insulin level. Poor nutrition reduces leptin and insulin levels in proportion to the decrease in body fat. A reduction in leptin and insulin levels then stimulates the hunger mechanism and leads to an increase in the hunger-producing hormones, e.g. neuropeptide Y (NPY) and Agouti-related peptide (AgRP).

A decrease in insulin and leptin levels also slows down the hunger-reducing mechanism and cuts the level of the hunger-reducing hormone Alpha-MSH. An increase in NPY and AgRP and the simultaneous reduction in Alpha-MSH in the hypothalamus causes the person to eat, i.e. ingest energy, and reduce their activity level, i.e. use less energy.

In late 1999, another new hormone, ghrelin, was discovered. It is produced in the wall of the stomach and increases with insufficient nutrition. A rise in ghrelin levels also stimulates the hunger-producing hormones NPY and AgRP. There is also a whole range of other known hormones whose functions are still unclear. Hormones produced in the intestines emit signals informing the hypothalamus about how full the digestive organs are and therefore also play a part in appetite regulation. [fig. 16]

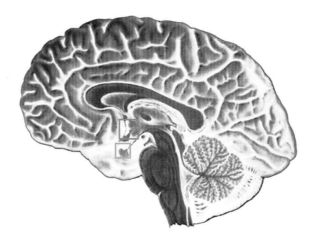

[Fig. 15] Cross-section through the brain along the central line, with the hypothalamus in the blue square and the pituitary gland in the red square.

weight. It is likely that their growth is controlled by other mechanisms in addition to growth hormone. However, there are clear grounds to suggest that the low level of growth hormone in PWS children is not simply a result of being overweight, but a genuine lack of growth hormone. This is suggested by the following:

Reduced Muscle Mass

In contrast to normal overweight children, children with PWS have low muscle mass.

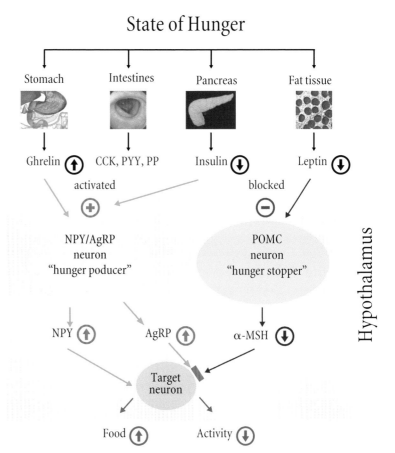

[Fig. 16] Incoming signals from the digestive tract and the fat tissue inform the hypothalamus on the nutritional status. The latter reacts by either producing a hunger feeling or satiety and an adaptation of activity (need for rest or movement). In PWS, this loop is disturbed (more information in the info box).

⊕ Increase
⊕ Decrease

Low IGF-I Level

Growth hormone produces linear growth mainly via another hormone, known as IGF-I, which is primarily produced in the liver. Despite a low level of growth hormone secretion, most overweight children produce normal or even high levels of IGF-I. Children with PWS, however, have low IGF-I levels. This indicates that PWS patients actually secrete a reduced amount of growth hormone.

Low Insulin Secretion

The low level of growth hormone secretion also explains the reduced insulin levels observed in children with PWS. In contrast, overweight children normally have high insulin levels. Low insulin secretion is typically found in children with a growth hormone deficiency.

Short Stature

The growth pattern of non-PWS overweight children differs from that of children with PWS. Most obese children are taller and grow more quickly than children with a normal weight. Children with PWS, conversely, are shorter and grow less rapidly than non-PWS children with a normal weight.

The growth hormone deficiency in children with PWS is probably caused by failure by the hypothalamus to regulate the secretion of the hormone correctly. In the early 1990s, long-term studies of growth hormone treatment for children with PWS were therefore launched in Europe and the USA. So far, results of treatment given for up to 7 years have been published. The figures produced by Aaron Carrel and his team in the USA, the Swedish study by Ann Lindgren and colleagues, and the study by the Zurich-based foundation 'Growth, Puberty, Adolescence' are particularly worthy of note. In most studies, growth hormone doses of around 1 mg/m^2 body surface area were given, which corresponds to approximately 0.025–0.05 mg/kg body weight/ day. Growth hormone not only promotes growth, but also increases muscle mass and reduces fat mass. [fig. 17 a/b]

Children with PWS grow significantly faster with growth hormone treatment; they develop more mucles and most either become or remain much less obese if the treatment is started very early. Parents also report that their children become more active within a few weeks of starting treatment, moving around more and with greater enjoyment. Fat mass decreases, but stabilises at a relatively high level. Meanwhile, muscle mass increases significantly in relation to body size during the first 6 months of growth hormone treatment. It then remains constant – still in relation to body size – and does not increase further through

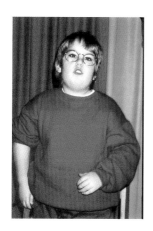 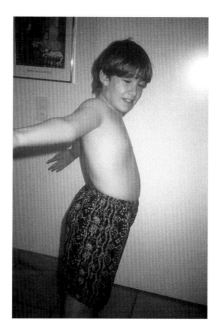

[Fig. 17 a/b] A child from the early phase of growth hormone treatment, before therapy and after two years of therapy. He rather impressively shows the success of a comprehensive management.

[Fig. 18 a/b] In this child too, strict control of food intake, combined with growth hormone treatment, led to considerable weight loss within one year.

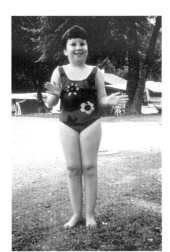

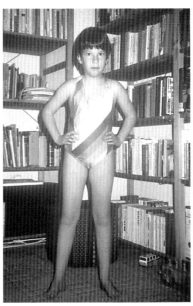

hormone treatment alone. However, since the children move around more because of their greater muscle strength, they build up their muscle mass.

Growth hormone treatment has fundamentally altered the outward appearance of PWS patients. For the first time ever, many children with PWS are no longer necessarily grossly over-weight – as long as calorie intake is properly controlled. [fig. 18 a/b]

Before parents opt for this therapy, they should certainly seek advice and take time over the decision. Growth hormone therapy requires perseverance: the daily injections have to be given for many years and a medical check-up is needed every 3–6 months.

Even when children with PWS receive growth hormone treatment, their appetite remains a problem and they still experience insatiable hunger. However, their fat mass and weight only fall if their energy intake does not rise. Even during growth hormone treatment, children with PWS can only avoid putting on weight if they keep their calorie intake at around 75% of the recommended level for healthy children. This means that eating must be monitored constantly even during such treatment.

What Are the Possible Side Effects and How Common Are They?

- Growth hormone counteracts the effects of insulin. Therefore, very overweight children in particular can suffer problems with their blood sugar metabolism. If a child receiving growth hormone therapy does not become slimmer or if their weight continues to increase in relation to their height, the child is clearly eating too much. However, a large increase in fatty tissue is the most common cause of blood sugar metabolism problems and can mean that treatment has to be stopped. If that is the case, the situation returns to normal in accordance with the child's body weight. Nevertheless, in less obese children with PWS, sugar metabolism is even improved in the long term during GH therapy, due to the uptake of sugar by the enhanced muscle mass.

- More rapid growth often inevitably leads to the aggravation of any existing scoliosis. Any curvature of the spine is therefore increased. However, this is not actually a side effect of growth hormone, but a direct consequence of growth – irrespective of whether the growth is completely natural or achieved through growth hormone injections. All children with PWS therefore need their spine to be checked regularly.

- A small proportion of children with PWS have respiratory problems, which perhaps can initially be made worse by growth hormone treatment. We therefore believe that each child's breathing should be monitored during their sleep by means of a polysomnograph or a similar method, especially before growth hormone treatment is offered. If anything is revealed, particularly if oxygen intake drops at times, caution should be exercised and the doctors concerned should think very carefully about how to proceed. In these circumstances, the tonsils are often enlarged. If they are removed, breathing is often either improved or fully restored to normal, so that growth hormone treatment may then be started.

Physical Exercise

Possibly due to the weakness of their muscles, motor development in babies with PWS is slow. In order to speed up their progress, parents and physiotherapists can do certain exercises with the baby. Because of their hypotonia and inadequate muscle

'Jeremy started growth hormone therapy when he was seven and a half. He had started school a few months before; his teacher did not know him very well, but she noticed the difference: he is now much more motivated, in PE he doesn't immediately complain about being tired, and he has started to do more things spontaneously. We quickly learned what to do with the injections and it wasn't long before Jeremy wanted to do them himself. He now injects himself some of the time in the hope that one day he will be as tall as his Dad.'

mass, these children need a kind of therapy similar to exercise in a fitness center. The aim of physiotherapy for babies with PWS is to increase their muscle mass. We adults know from our own experience that this is an exhausting and arduous process.

PWS children are generally too quiet and too sedentary. Their muscles are underdeveloped mainly because they do not move around enough. It is therefore important to encourage babies to move and exercise more. Although it may be hard for the parents, it is helpful if they repeatedly put their child in body positions that they do not like so that they feel uncomfortable and begin to struggle and cry. This increases their activity level

'Monika started physiotherapy when she was 5 months old because she could not lift her head on her own. Every step had to be worked at really hard. Monika also received occupational therapy as part of her remedial education programme.'

'In the first two years, we took Jeremy to the physiotherapist four times a week and, of course, he practised more at home! We then took a year off, firstly to take a break from the endless visits to the children's hospital, and secondly, with the paediatrician's support, to see how Jeremy would develop on his own. Then we started the physiotherapy again once a week, together with weekly visits to an occupational therapist to help with his fine motor skills.'

and is the best form of muscle training. We think that the Vojta method of physiotherapy is particularly suitable for babies with PWS. The Vojta technique is a special form of physiotherapy in which the babies are put into various body positions which are designed to increase their muscle activity (www.vojta.com).

Older children also tend to dislike movement. However, most PWS children have fairly good fine motor skills. This means that they are happy to sit and play, but do not romp around as much as other children of the same age. Motivational games and physiotherapeutic support with corresponding movement training can help to increase their desire to move around. The child's sense of balance needs to be developed as well as their muscles and this can be achieved through play, for example using roller skates.

As with all therapies, it is important – and very difficult – to find the right level where motor skills development is concerned. The child should be pushed to comply, but not be asked to do much more than it is capable of. It is often hard for parents to decide how much specialist training, in addition to all their efforts to improve their other various skills, they can and should expect their child to undergo at the same time still allowing them time to simply be children. [fig. 19]

Many parents whose children had been given growth hormone treatment noticed that the therapy had a positive influence and the children felt like moving around more than before. However, even with such treatment, children with PWS move significantly less than healthy children. In a research project carried out by the Zurich-based foundation 'Growth, Puberty, Adolescence', the spontaneous physical activity of PWS children undergoing growth hormone therapy was measured using pedometers. Pedometers convert motion impulses into distances and show the result in kilometers. Children with PWS and a control sample of healthy children each wore a pedometer for 3 consecutive days. We noted that children with PWS managed only 11 km in 3 days,

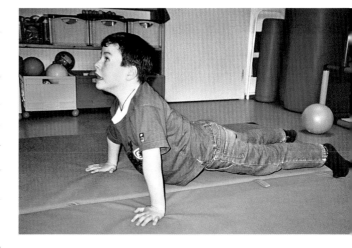

[Fig. 19] A 6-year-old with PWS during his training exercises during physiotherapy.

whereas children in the control group covered 26 km. Despite receiving growth hormone treatment, children with PWS therefore show a definite aversion to physical activity. This so-called hypoactivity is just as significant as the constant feeling of hunger.

The next stage of the study looked at whether the muscles of children with PWS can be trained in the same way as those of healthy children. To this end, we devised an exercise for the strengthening of the lower leg muscles, to be carried out for 3–4 minutes each day for a period of 3 months. Thanks to this exercise, the muscle mass in the lower legs of PWS children increased significantly and reached the maximum level after about 50 days of training on average. A similar pattern was found in healthy children. It therefore seems to be possible to increase the muscle mass of PWS patients at the same rate as that of healthy children. We can therefore conclude that the reduced muscle mass of PWS children is a direct consequence of their lack of physical activity.

It was also very gratifying to discover that by the end of the training programme, the PWS children showed a significant increase in spontaneous physical activity. Their daily walking distance rose from 45 to 70% of that of the control group. This means that it is possible to improve the behavior pattern of PWS children who mainly play in a sitting position by using a simple 3-minutes-a-day exercise programme.

The researchers also measured the children's physical abilities at the beginning, end and 3 months after the end of the exercise programme. It emerged that for both groups, i.e. PWS children and the healthy control sample, the exercise programme resulted in a significant improvement in physical ability. Some children with PWS almost trebled their performance levels while the healthy children in the control group had at least doubled

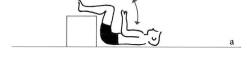

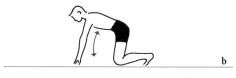

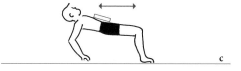

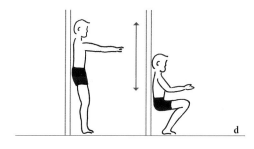

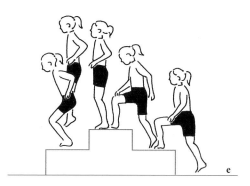

[Fig. 20] Physical training programme for children with PWS (5–10 minutes, if possible every day):

a 'Jack-knife exercise' (abdominal muscles): supine position, upper legs in a right-angle position to the body, lower legs horizontally and supported by a chair, lift the upper part of the body until the bell is reached.

b Push-ups on the knees (breast and arm muscles): on all fours, lower the upper body until touching the floor with the nose tip.

c Upside-down four-legged walk (arm and buttocks muscles): on all fours, belly showing upwards and the back facing the floor, walk forward and backward through the room. This exercise is best performed while carrying a cushion on the belly, which should not fall down.

d 'Sitting against the wall' (thigh muscles): stand with the back at the wall, lower the upper body into a sitting position, without the bottom being supported by a chair. Maintain this position for as long as possible.

e Climbing stairs (leg muscles): climb two steps and jump down the steps one after another, thereby pushing off and landing smoothly, cushioning body weight.

theirs by the end of the programme. Once the special programme was finished, the physical abilities of both groups dropped, but remained higher than when the study began, which suggests that the exercise programme may have a long-term effect.

We were therefore able to show that a short exercise programme carried out regularly for around three minutes per day is sufficient to drastically improve local muscle mass and the level of spontaneous physical activity. [fig. 20]

Parents and carers of children with PWS must be made aware of the importance of physical activity. Each PWS patient needs a personal exercise programme adapted to their age and respective interests and abilities, taking 3–4 minutes each day. This new approach to the treatment of PWS represents another important form of therapy, alongside controlled eating and growth hormone treatment.

Sex Hormone Therapy

Controlled by the hypothalamus, the pituitary gland secretes two hormones which in turn control the sex glands – the testes in boys and ovaries in girls. In healthy males, the testes are already active before birth and produce hormones which are involved, inter alia, in ensuring that the testes descend from the stomach into the scrotum. Later on, at the instigation of the pituitary gland, the sex hormones produced in the testes and ovaries trigger pubertal development. This begins on average at age 11 for girls and 13 for boys. After puberty, the hormone produced in the testes (testosterone) is responsible for sexual desire and virility. The same role is played in women by the hormones produced in the ovaries (estrogen and progesterone), which also control the menstrual cycle.

When they first described PWS, Prader, Willi and Labhart noted that, to some extent at least, the testes or ovaries of the children they had examined were probably not properly regulated. In boys, this phenomenon is evident after birth in the fact that their testes have not descended from the stomach to the scrotum while in the womb and that their penis is small. The lack of pubertal development is another later indication. In girls, it is evident in their undersized small lips of the vulva, and they also sometimes do not experience pubertal development. Many do not have periods.

It is still unclear whether and when undescended testes are damaged. Child hormone experts, however, believe that undescended testes should be moved into the scrotum before a child's second birthday, so that they can be protected from possible damage. Of course, this operation may also be carried out later in life. If a boy with PWS is subsequently treated with the

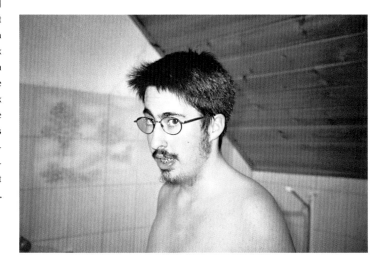

[Fig. 21] An adolescent with PWS, treated with growth hormone and sex hormones. Apart from the increase of muscle mass, male sex hormones lead to change of voice, the facial traits take on more distinctively male characteristics and the adolescent starts to grow a beard.

male hormone testosterone at the onset of puberty, the testes may, as a result of the higher hormone level, descend into the scrotum themselves. The decision whether undescended testes in boys with PWS should be moved into the scrotum early in life is therefore often tricky in individual cases.

Whether the missing sex hormones should be replaced is still a controversial question. Experts have differing opinions on the matter. However, it is clear that even disabled children have a right to normal pubertal development, for this is also an important social process. A regular menstrual cycle can help young women, for example, to feel like normal, adult women. The same applies to young men, for whom a deep voice, masculine facial features and body and facial hair can generate greater self-confidence. [fig. 21]

One side effect of the pubertal development of PWS patients, particularly males, can be a deterioration of psychological sensitivity and more frequent fits of rage and stubbornness. It is therefore useful to discuss with the doctor in detail whether and when sex hormone treatment should be started. It is important to remember that, if it causes major problems, such treatment can be interrupted at any time.

Sex hormone therapy is administered to girls and boys in different ways. Girls are given a pill containing female hormones such as the contraceptive pill, but without the contraceptive effect. This is impossible with boys since, taken in pill form, the male sex hormones would be inactivated by the liver before they take effect. The hormones are therefore usually given in an injection every 4 weeks, with doses given by a doctor in accordance with the patient's age and stage of development.

Developmental Support

The earlier potential developmental problems are spotted, the more likely it is that the child, with the help of supportive and corrective measures, will be able to develop its abilities. It is therefore important that attention is paid at an early stage to any possible deviations from the norm in children with PWS. The

'Stefan developed his own language, which for a long time could barely be understood, even by those closest to him. Since he turned five, he has been to a speech therapist as well as a physio-therapist. When he was four, he went to a weekly play group and now, at five, he is in a special needs nursery school. He is then expected to move to a special needs school, where he will continue to receive individual support.'

pediatrician may therefore monitor the child more regularly than normal. Clinical examinations, tests and, above all, parental observation can unearth information about potential deficiencies and provide an early indication that certain supportive therapies are necessary.

The development of intelligence and learning skills also varies among children with PWS; learning abilities are usually moderately impaired. Even shortly after birth, a child's parents can promote their development by stimulating them with music, language, mobiles over the cot, games, etc. This is particularly important because PWS children are quiet babies who cry less and are less curious about their environment than other children – which is why they need more stimulation. At this age, it is mainly a case of early stimulation and physiotherapy.

Later on, speech development problems are to the fore. Up to 1 in 3 children with PWS have serious difficulties in learning to talk; regular speech therapy sessions are very helpful. Some countries are also experimenting with a different strategy, where children with PWS are taught sign language as well as speech. This enables them to express some of their wishes and thoughts very precisely at an earlier stage.

Often, children with PWS are selectively gifted, i.e. they have strengths and weaknesses in different branches of learning. Their understanding of language is usually more advanced than their speaking ability. It is important to recognise the deficiencies and abilities of each individual child and to offer support in problem areas – and to offer praise when they do well. Specialist help is usually necessary. Intelligence should be tested in specialist centers to which GPs can refer PWS patients.

It is vital that the strengths and weaknesses of children with PWS should be identified before they start school because, depending on what kind of education is chosen, the child's learning ability may be suitably stretched or possibly overstretched. Many children with PWS feel most comfortable in small classes which can be better tailored to their individual learning speed. However, there is no rule of thumb here and parents must decide, in consultation with nursery and schoolteachers, remedial education specialists, doctors, psychologists and other experts, which route is best for their child.

Psychological Support

Restricting energy intake and increasing energy consumption are the most important tasks for carers of children with PWS. In most cases, the parents must take the responsibility for this. They must control their child's desire to eat 24 hours a day and motivate their child to carry out a clearly defined exercise pro-

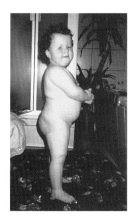
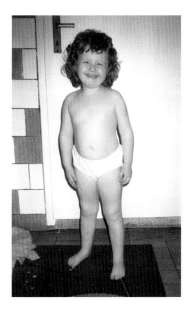

[Fig. 22 a/b] Loss of weight exclusively thanks to a strict monitoring of food intake. The difference between the two pictures is a 30-minute telephone consultation with the physician and two years of strict eating control.

gramme – and that in a child who is likely to be difficult and display behavioral problems. [fig. 22 a/b]

Living with a PWS child is often very hard, requiring parents to be very strong and often to sacrifice their own ambitions and priorities. We have found, for example, that mothers of children with PWS are much less likely to work than mothers of healthy children. Closer questioning has shown that they are usually unable to work because their child takes up all their en-

'We had to choose between a normal class, a special remedial class or class C, a small class for children with speech or sensory disorders. After much thought, we opted for class C. So far, we parents and Monika are happy with that choice. Monika's favourite subject is reading, but she also enjoys writing and arithmetic. She joins in the PE lessons, but rather cautiously. She has devised some clever strategies for getting out of it – for example, she enjoys being the referee in games.'

ergy and resources. Yet the resources of parents with PWS children are not inexhaustible – they often feel exhausted, worn out and as if they have no strength or patience left. How can they deal with this situation? What should they do when their son demands food virtually every minute, when he has another tantrum and refuses to go to school? Dear parents, remember you are not alone. There are numerous professional advisers, psychologists and psychiatrists, who can come alongside you to help – and even show you ways out of seemingly impossible situations. It is often important to learn how to improve the way you divide your strength and resources and not to be ashamed of seeking professional help.

Since children and adults with PWS are more likely to have psychological problems than other people, the use of various psychiatric drugs, including tranquillisers, has been tested. The tranquilliser sold in the USA under the name Prozac, for example, has been mentioned in relation to PWS; this is a kind of lifestyle drug which is said to have amazing results. However, a critical scientific study has shown that Prozac is no more or less effective than other similar tranquillisers. No psychiatric drug is especially suitable for PWS. If such drugs are necessary, the psychiatrist responsible will prescribe the same medication as he would for a patient without PWS who shows the same symptoms. It is important to remember, however, that PWS patients usually react much more strongly to such medication. Their dose should therefore be determined very carefully.

There are therefore no wonder drugs which can solve all the psychological problems of people with PWS. Nor is there a miracle appetite suppressant. The same therefore applies to people with PWS as to others: every situation should be assessed individually in consultation with the relevant doctor and medicinal treatment should be considered very carefully.

Upbringing

We have investigated the educational methods used by families of children with PWS and compared them with those of a control group of families with healthy children. Parents of PWS children were much more consistent in the way they brought up their children than those of the control group – and not just in relation to eating. They also punished their children less.

The study also showed, in simplified terms, a direct relationship between parents' educational methods and the weight of PWS children. A consistent upbringing helps to keep weight at a reasonable level. In the control group families – those without PWS – there was no such correlation, since the energy balance of healthy children with a normal weight does not require any external control. Of course, there are huge differences between individual cases. However, in general it seems that the educational methods used by parents of PWS children are very important. In the field of energy regulation in particular, the demands made on parents are nevertheless often virtually impossible. They should therefore not be afraid to seek psychological support in the form of educational counselling.

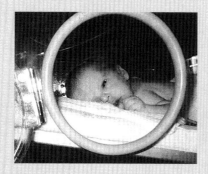
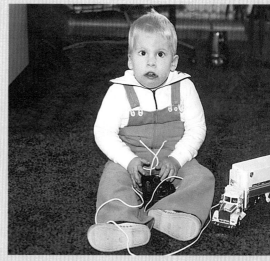
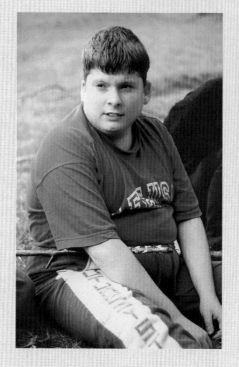
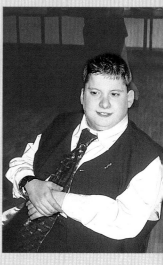

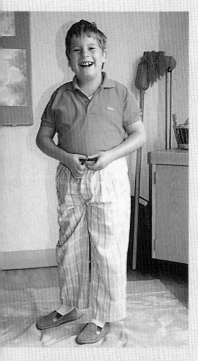

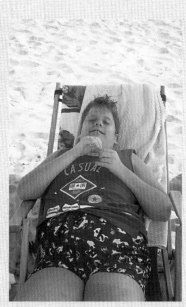

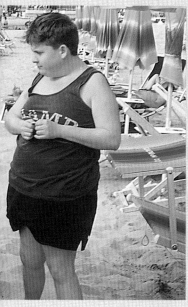

Piero

Piero is a typical example for the development of a PWS child that does not receive consistent care and growth hormone therapy. A typical element is the need for a gastric feeding tube, early weight increase and a behaviour which leads to the accumulation of energy reserves. These pictures show that the children affected, apart from eating too much, try to avoid moving as much as possible. Most of the time, they simply sit or lie around.

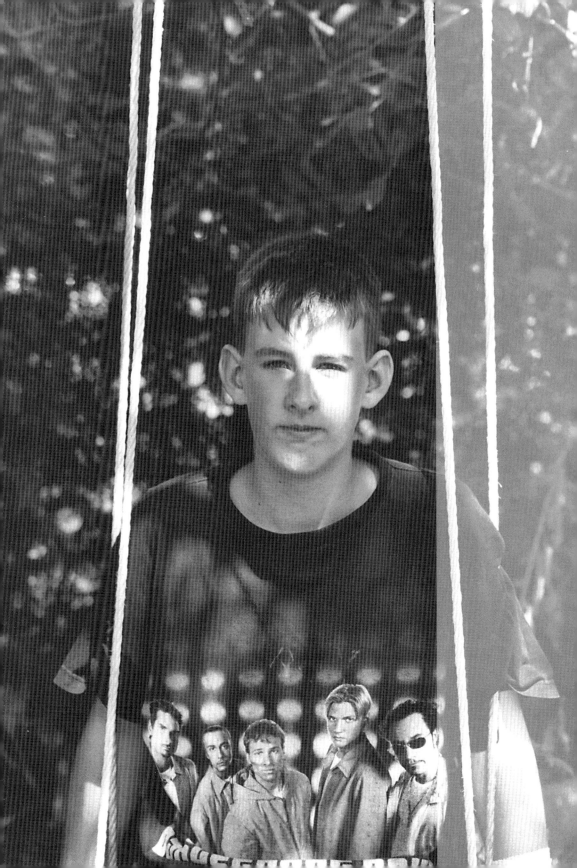

Concluding Remarks

'I believe the most important thing is to accept the child for what he or she is. A PWS child is and always will be disabled. However, the calmer the parents are with their disabled child, the fewer "typical" PWS problems will arise. Nothing is worse than careless, inconsistent parents. The child should be stretched, but not overstretched.'

Of course, much more could be said and reported about PWS: things that parents have experienced and discovered through living with a child with PWS, strategies for dealing with school authorities, health insurance companies, brothers and sisters of PWS children, and other family members. A booklet like this is not enough. Neither can it meet all the personal needs related to PWS: neighbors, friends, relatives, teachers and therapists have a huge variety of questions; parents need advice, particularly in difficult situations such as when PWS is first diagnosed. And PWS patients themselves obviously have practical needs of their own.

Since this booklet is primarily intended as an information guide for people with no experience of PWS, it is likely that many parents will, quite understandably, feel that it does not adequately meet their needs in their specific situation. Here, therefore, to conclude is a word of advice from a mother of a child with PWS to all parents of PWS children:

'Use the self-help group, make contact with other parents. Together we are strong and can achieve much. For me personally, it has particularly helped me to:

- cope with the idea of having a disabled child,
- find comfort when yet another situation seems hopeless,
- find the right therapies and therapists for my child,
- find help with dealing with the authorities,
- be involved in making people more aware of PWS and bringing it to the attention of doctors, therapists and experts,
- find people to talk to who are going through similar things as we are with our child, and, finally, the children themselves also enjoy doing things together as a group!' [fig. 23]

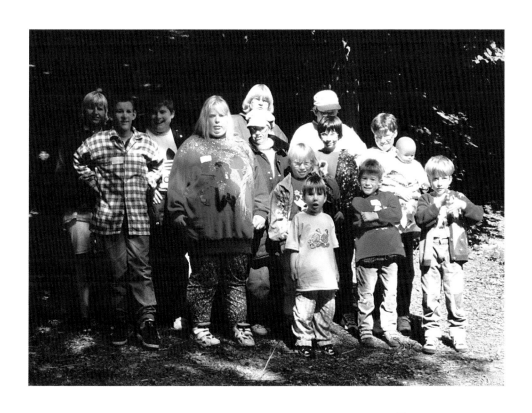

[Fig. 23] PWS children of two different generations: with and without comprehensive management.

Addresses and Websites of
National and International Parents' Associations

Switzerland

Swiss PWS Association

Andreas Bächli (President)

Bugg 3

CH–9478 Azmoos

E-mail: mail@prader-willi.ch

www.prader-willi.ch

Austria

Österreichische Gesellschaft Prader-Willi Syndrom Selbsthilfegruppe von Betroffenen für Betroffene

Dr. phil. Verena Wanker-Gutmann

Schloss Frohnburg, Hellbrunner Allee 53

AT–5020 Salzburg

E-mail: frohnburg@salzburg.co.at

www.prader-willi-syndrom.at

Germany

Prader Willi Syndrom Vereinigung Deutschland e.V.

Thomas Groß (Chairman)

Söllockweg 66

DE–45357 Essen

E-mail: ThomasGross@prader-willi.de

www.prader-willi.de

France

Association Prader-Willi France

Jean-Yves Belliard (President)

10, rue Charles Clément

FR–02500 Mondrepuis

E-mail: jean-yves.belliard@wanadoo.fr

http://perso.wanadoo.fr/pwillifr

Italy

Federazione delle Associazioni Italiane per l'aiuto ai soggetti con sindrome Prader-Willi

Maria Antonietta Ricci (President)

Via Manzoni 29/b

IT–10040 Druento

E-mail: apwto@tin.it

www.dedalus.it/prader-willi

UK

Prader-Willi Syndrome Association (UK)

125a London Road

Derby DE1 2QQ

England

E-mail: Website@pwsa-uk.demon.co.uk

www.pwsa-uk.demon.co.uk/index.htm

USA

Prader-Willi Syndrome Association (USA)

Janalee Heinemann (Executive Director)

5700 Midnight Pass Road, Suite 6

Sarasota, FL 34242

E-mail: execdir@pwsausa.org

www.pwsausa.org

International PWS Association

Pam Eisen (President)

E-mail: pam@ipwso.org

www.ipwso.org

Further information and literature can be found at: www.childgrowth.org